Herbs & Supplements for College Students

~ The Best Herbs & Supplements to Increase Energy, Support Focus for Extended Periods of Studying, & Maximize Memory & Retention of New Information ~

Patrick Devlin

Copyright © 2016 Patrick Devlin

All rights reserved.

ISBN-10: 1536876100
ISBN-13: 978-1536876109

DEDICATION

This book is dedicated to my sister Katie: thank you for your encouragement in my writings!

Disclosures

No statement in this book has been evaluated by the Food and Drug Administration. No products are intended to diagnose, treat, cure, or prevent any disease.

I do not receive any royalties, stipends, or compensation for promoting any product in this book. In all cases where I recommend a specific product, it is because I believe that is the best product available.

By reading this book, you agree that if you are taking any prescription medication(s), have a pre-existing medical or psychological condition, are taking over-the-counter drugs, or are taking any other supplements, that you will consult with your doctor and with a pharmacist before taking any supplements I recommend in this book.

CONTENTS

1	Understand This Book	1
2	The 'Four Groups'	2
3	Supplements for Energy	3-15
4	Supplements for Depression	16-19
5	Supplements for Addiction	20-25
6	Supplements to Avoid	26-29
7	Supplements for Illnesses	30-36
8	Creating a Supplement Stack	37-42
9	For Additional Reading	43-47
10	Bibliography	48-50

ACKNOWLEDGMENTS

This book would not have been possible without my sister Katie encouraging me to write whenever she can, thank you for the encouragement Katie!

Also, I am very grateful to a good friend, Rev. David Martin whom I met whilst he was studying in the Bay Area and who encouraged me throughout my studies at the University of California, Davis.

UNDERSTAND THIS BOOK

This book is intended for college students who are struggling with extremely busy schedules, but who are having difficulty keeping up with the work required.

My Goals Throughout This Book:

- Short & Concise. No 20-page chapters.

- The best supplements for energy and memory only.

- I will never try to get you to start some new diet.

- I only recommend specific brands because I have researched them. I do not work for any company, nor do I receive money for promoting specific companies

- I will tell you supplements that work, not explain their history. Simple is better.

- *This is not a book on herbal medicine*: I recommend supplements that are both herbal and chemical.

If this sounds good, let's get started!

2 ~ THE "4 GROUPS"

Every college student has different problems with which they struggle, and supplements and other *easy and basic* changes can help exponentially and make you gain a huge advantage in your studies.

The "Top 4" Issues:
Lack of Energy
Low Motivation
Focus Issues
Remembering What You Learn

In this part of the book, I will briefly describe supplements you can take that will directly benefit your studies. I will also describe non-supplemental methods to help with these issues.

Feelings of Despair & Depression
In this part of the book, I will explain which supplements and other methods you can use to help you cope with (and overcome!) these awful feelings.

Overcome/Prevent: Hangovers & Drug Use
I will explain some of the best ways to overcome hangovers and drug withdrawals, and I will explain methods you can use to help with your overall health.

Get Over the Flu, Stomach Flu, & Common Cold
Among the things that most impact your studies, being sick is just not a fun thing to deal with. I will give you a list of supplements and lifestyle practices so that you get back to peak health quickly.

INCREASE ENERGY AND MOTIVATION
&
INCREASE FOCUS AND REMEMBERING WHAT YOU LEARN

In this section, I will give you the fastest ways you can increase both your mental energy and your physical energy.

I will also give you the best ways to increase your motivation, for if you are highly motivated, you will be driven to accomplish so much more.

CORDYCEPS

Cordyceps are an interesting supplement that if you choose to take only them and nothing else recommended in this book, you would see an definite change in your overall health. Cordyceps are an important part of Traditional Chinese Medicine, but Cordyceps are listed as an endangered fungus in China, so they are grown on rice for commercial use.

> Cordyceps are the best supplement for increasing energy. If you only take one supplement, take Cordyceps.

Cordyceps are made up of Cordycepin (3' deoxyadenosine), ergosterol, polysaccharides, a glycoproteins, and peptides with α-aminoisobutyric acid, which gives immunomodulatory, anti-oxidant, anti-inflammatory, neuroprotective, and many other effects. (Paterson, 1474).

Avoid all proprietary formulas you find for Cordyceps supplements, most do not work well, if at all. I recommend these three brands:

NOW Foods Cordyceps
Dragon Herbs Cordyceps
Host Defense Cordyceps

There are other good brands, but these are the ones I found to be most useful. Interestingly, Dragon Herbs has a product called 'Munchable Cordyceps' if you're interested in trying that, but it is frequently out of stock.

Overall, one of the best supplements a student can take. Very highly recommended.

LION'S MANE

The Lion's Mane mushroom contains β-glucan polysaccharides which give it a number of good qualities, among them immune system boosting effects, but most importantly, the ability to activate your Nerve Growth Factor or NGF.

People's brains stop growing when they are around 25 and from there on out, they start losing millions of brain cells daily, increased to hundreds of millions of brain cells if they drink even small amounts of alcohol or are in a toxic environment with pollution or if they get an autoimmune disease. What the Lion's Mane mushroom does is that it does not directly reverse this, but instead it starts brain cells growing so that you get some of them back. This is especially noticeable in elderly people with Alzheimer's who have nearly lost all of their ability to remember anything. After starting Lion's Mane supplementation (which takes a month to a half year for effects to be noticed), they have surprised their caregivers by starting to remember things again.

Obviously, for students, this is extremely useful since students often eat a poor diet, but even with the best diet in the world, more brain cells equals better grades in classes, so this is a supplement I recommend all students take.

I recommend the "Host Defense – Lion's Mane" product as it is high quality. One gram of Lion's Mane a day will help you exponentially. Just remember, you won't see results immediately. But… I *guarantee* you will see results eventually, so do not stop taking these.

BRAINWAVE ENTRAINMENT

Brainwave Entrainment or BWE has been known of since the late 1800s, or more recently known of as Binaural Beats. More recently, Isochronic Tones, a newer generation of Binaural Beats were created, yet both Binaural Beats and Isochronic Tones are equally effective.

Binaural Beats work by playing different frequencies of sound into each of your ears, and thus, a good quality pair of headphones is required, speakers simply will not work. This causes your brainwaves to attune to the difference in sound frequencies and alters your mood accordingly. Isochronic Tones are similar, but they work by playing a certain tone at regular intervals, so while you don't need headphones, I strongly recommend still wearing them.

There are a lot of very low quality soundtracks available, so I will recommend a few of my favorites. All you will need is a good quality of headphones (you won't notice much with earbuds, headphones are pretty much required).

Binaural/Isochronic Tracks I Recommend:
https://youtu.be/RYDUQx0iIN4

https://youtu.be/1Ryh4v40l0s

Both of these examples I listed are *excellent* tracks. It is important to listen to the entire track (it takes time for your brainwaves to readjust to a different state). You should wear headphones, and, ideally, close your eyes (trust me, you won't fall asleep).

I really have found Jason Lewis's tracks to be the most useful, but there are many Binaural or Isochronic tracks on YouTube or elsewhere. Many are not quite as effective, so I recommend sticking to ones produced by Jason Lewis.

PIRACETAM

Piracetam is a very interesting supplement that helps significantly in boosting energy and in the formation of new memories (which is perfect for students who have much to remember!). It is under the brand name Nootropil in Europe, but the FDA has forbidden its use as a drug or supplement. In Mexico, the pharmaceutical giant GlaxoSmithKline makes it under a brand name.

However, in the US, due to the lack of FDA approval, Piracetam can be freely sold (alongside labels denoting it is not intended for human consumption). Just ignore these labels, for Piracetam is very safe. I get Piracetam from the Peak Nootropics website, but there are many versions available.

Piracetam affects the neurotransmitter acetylcholine via the ACh receptors, which is important in the memory process (Winnicka), and thus it has gained a huge user base among students. Because it uses choline through its mechanism of action, you should make sure you get a good source of choline. I recommend not taking a choline supplement since they are notorious for not being too precise. I recommend instead eating one hardboiled egg for each gram of Piracetam you take. I recommend starting with 0.5g a day and building up to 3-5g a day over two weeks.

One gram is roughly ¼ teaspoon of Piracetam powder. Mix it into a glass of water, and I recommend pinching your nose and drinking it quickly. Have something to eat after drinking it, for it is one of the most bitter things I've ever tasted. But it works extremely well, so it is absolutely worth it, and it is extremely safe. Highly recommended. Just don't forget 1 hardboiled egg per gram of Piracetam (or you'll get a splitting headache). Cooked chicken is also a source of choline. One of the best of the best study supplements.

GINSENG

American Ginseng ~ *excellent*
This is an excellent supplement students can take, I like the NOW Foods one, but honestly any product is good as long as it isn't too expensive and is well-reviewed on Amazon. American Ginseng is best for people who feel tired frequently, since it acts strongly against fatigue.

Korean Ginseng ~ *good*
Korean ginseng is good, but it is heavily marketed as a sex supplement, which is mostly marketing, so I'd stick with American ginseng. I generally try to steer people in the direction of American ginseng because it has a stronger stimulating effect, but Korean ginseng is known for supporting a 'natural' feeling of energy. Worth trying, but if you're in a hurry, just go with a quality American ginseng supplement.

Panax Ginseng / Chinese Ginseng ~ *avoid*
Not recommended. People either report good or bad effects. It doesn't help me, personally, at all. Many products on the market rave about all the antioxidants in it (because they aren't able to rave about its energy boosting effects because it doesn't have many).

~ ~ ~

Ginseng is one of those supplements with which I recommend exercising extreme caution as to which company you purchase it from unless it is grown in the United States (eg. American Ginseng), for Ginseng – especially Chinese Ginseng – is known for contamination with toxins like lead. Companies like NOW Foods or Dragon Herbs are trustworthy, but choose quality here.

ENERGY DRINKS

Highly Recommended Energy Drinks:
- Guayaki Traditional Tereré (cold-brewed Yerba Mate leaves with added sugar)
- Root 9 (Korean Ginseng-based energy drinks)

Acceptable Energy Drinks:
- Starbucks Double Shot
- Coffee-based energy drinks (with no added ingredients except sugar, milk, flavors, gum, etc.)
- MEGs (Military Energy Gum) – purchasable on amazon.com, each piece of gum contains 100mg of caffeine but also contains both aspartame and sucralose, neither of which is good for your body. Interestingly, nicotine absorbs through your mouth's membranes within minutes whereas energy drinks take roughly 30 minutes for the caffeine to get into your bloodstream.

Avoid at All Costs:
- Most brand-name energy drinks (eg. Monster, Redbull, Rockstar, Redline, Amp, etc.) – they contain lots of ingredients who stimulate you for about 30 minutes to 1 hour and afterwards remain in your liver and consume your precious energy while your body attempts to detox.
- Caffeine pills (never take these, they're terrible for your body and don't work very well). If you must, take the MEGs I mentioned above.
- Proprietary formulas of "energy boosting" supplements from various companies like NOW foods.
- Any pre-workout supplement with caffeine in it.
- Energy drinks with added B vitamins, taurine, guarana, or anything else you can't pronounce.

WHAT'S WRONG WITH _____?

I recommend *avoiding* any supplement with added:
- Taurine
- Guarana
- Aspartame
- Sucralose
- Stevia
- Corn Syrup
- High Fructose Corn Syrup
- Any Acid other than Citric Acid (eg. Phosphoric Acid in Pepsi)
- Creatine
- BCAAs
- CoQ-10
- Greater than 20g sugar per 16 fl oz.
- Carrageenan

Why do I recommend avoiding these things? Especially when I mentioned the latest supplemental 'god,' Stevia, I suspect you raised your eyebrows. In this book, I urge you to *not* take anything that will *fool* your body, instead take things that *help* your body. A small amount of sugar will not hurt you, but corn syrup instead of sugar adds a degree of uncertainty to your life: how was the corn syrup manufactured? What quality was it? And so on. Citric Acid is an alternative name for Vitamin C, Phosphoric Acid is an alternative name for 'teeth destroyer.'

You may take the following:
- Tea, coffee, herbs/herb extracts
- Low added sugar/no sugar added
- Citric acid, flavoring, electrolyte ingredients

POWER NAP

A power nap uses knowledge of the length of circadian rhythm to its use, and times a nap so that you feel rested after a very short time of sleep. While scientists don't know the exact mechanism as to how sleep helps, what is known is that when you sleep, your brain heals any injuries sustained during the day, and, most importantly, processes new information you learned the previous day.

A good length for a power nap is 25-45 minutes (and even if you cannot fall asleep, simply lying down and closing your eyes for this length of time can have excellent effects). What you are doing is giving your brain a quick reset, which clears your thoughts and gives you a boost for further studies. Never fall into the trap of listening to music, having a TV or any of the like.

Increasingly popular recently are 'night modes' on phones, where the blue wavelength is reduced, and the screen has a distinctively yellow color. While it may be a little annoying at the start, this is excellent, for the blue wavelength (think laptop screensaver, smartphone, etc.) stimulates your brain for up to an hour after looking at it, so you should avoid blue night lamps, blue screens, etc., in order to fall asleep more quickly. An exception to the music rule is you might consider listening to an Isochronic or Binaural soundtrack with some headphones while you are taking a power nap, again, I recommend Jason Lewis's soundtracks on YouTube, but there are many others available.

The main key for a power nap is do not sleep longer than 45 minutes or you will enter deep sleep, where you will feel groggy when you awaken instead of refreshed. A power nap is a powerful tool that you should definitely make use of.

WATER

Often overlooked in the frantic hours of studying or cramming for a test is a glass of water. This can have devastating effects on your energy and focus, for caffeine is dehydrating and when studying, your brain is more active and thus you study better.

On a side note, when studying attempt to find a quiet and *cool* place. When you are hot, your body is sweating and trying to eliminate the heat through sweat, so a cool place like a library is excellent.

Remember, even though water makes you need to use the restroom more frequently, a well-hydrated brain functions better, helps prevent fatigue, helps with studies, and helps your immune system keep you from becoming sick.

Overall, a few large glasses of water throughout the day, even when you are not thirsty, are often enough to help give you that extra boost of energy.

GYNOSTEMMA TEA

Gynostemma tea has maintained popularity all through China for several decades as a so-called 'longevity' boosting tea, for Gynostemma is a grass that grows in China and is dried and used as tea.

It is, at best, a mild non-stimulating stimulant (which makes it excellent if you need to stay awake and study and also excellent to relax your mind just before you go to bed).

The best way to describe the feeling of a cup of Gynostemma tea is if you think of the feeling of opening a window in a warm house and feeling a breath of fresh air coming in through the window.

This tea has that effect: it is a mild awakening feeling, so do not except any powerful effects, but instead expect a feeling of calm, yet alertness.

You can buy this tea on Amazon.com or most specialty health food stores, and my on preference is the Dragon Herbs one from Amazon.com, but as this tea is so famous throughout China, there are many options available.

ADRAFINIL

Adrafinil is a 'pro drug' or a nootropic, and as you can guess from the diagram to the left, this is not derived from any plant or 'natural' substance but is, instead, a chemical that is cooked up in a laboratory. This is completely legal in the United States, so don't get the wrong impression, I recommend Peak Nootropics but there are many sites from which you can purchase this.

Adrafinil is a powerful drug that will basically delete any feeling of fatigue from your brain for a long period of time (roughly 5-8 hours). It is not so much a focusing drug, but rather if you are extremely tired, you feel like you slept for hours (even though you did not). Adrafinil is metabolized in your liver into Modafinil (which is a prescription-only drug in the US) but because Adrafinil is not Modafinil until it gets to your liver, it is currently unscheduled (read 'legal'). This being said, you will likely wake up the next morning with a very fatigued feeling, so I recommend closing off your studies with 500mg or so of Milk Thistle to help your liver detox itself.

Adrafinil should be considered a very useful supplement for procrastinators. It is often accompanied with stomach pain, but if you are at the point where caffeine does not help, Adrafinil, I assure you: will help. Remember to take Milk Thistle before bed, though, so that you will feel better the next day.

GMOs

This is where I will explain to you why it is dangerous for you to avoid any product containing GMOs. No, you read that correctly, this book makes no secret of the fact that I'm not on a mission to shove some weird diet or philosophy down your throat.

GMOs (or Genetically Modified Organisms) sounds scary and probably brings up vague thoughts of what friends of yours may have said about companies like Monsanto or rumors of super-weeds or other harmful things. Genetically modified food is... let's just say... 100% of the food you eat: half of which is genetically modified the 'natural' way by hybridization and farming techniques and half of which is genetically modified in a laboratory.

GMOs are subject to intense government scrutiny and undergo rigorous testing that verifies they are safe for humans, do not cause cancer or allergies, and many other criteria. The so-called 'natural' alternatives (namely, conventional or organic food) does not undergo any testing and is subject to very little (if any) government oversight beyond the minimum. So if you want to eat something that is the best for your health, I would recommend you eat products that contain GMOs, if this is not available, eat organic food, and avoid conventionally grown food.

If you're looking for a good video on this subject, watch the following video: https://www.youtube.com/watch?v=aA4I-WRu_s0

OVERCOMING DEPRESSION & DESPAIR & BECOMING CONFIDENT

In this section, I will give you the fastest ways you can overcome depression and despair and become more confident than you ever thought you could be.

ST. JOHN'S WORT

St. John's Wort is the best supplement you can take if you are struggling with feelings of worthlessness, depression, or chronic fatigue.

> St. John's Wort is the best supplement you can take if you feel depressed or hopeless. It will get you back on your feet. I highly recommend good quality tinctures over cheaper pills, you want quality over price for this supplement.

It is very important that you understand that if you take any medication with an SSRI, that you do not take St. John's Wort, as the two have a major interaction with each other which can lead to something called 'serotonin syndrome' which may require hospitalization.

Taken by itself though, St. John's Wort is one of the most critical things you can do to change your life around. Understand that you will no longer be able to drink alcohol heavily, but you will no longer want to anyway.

St. John's Wort is hard to cultivate so often manufacturers will dilute it down to a very weak formula, so this is not a supplement you want to buy for the cheapest price you can find. Look for a quality supplement with good reviews on Amazon.com or, better still, talk to a specialist at a local health store and purchase what they recommend.

CANNABIDIOL (CBD)

Cannabidiol is an invaluable resource for anyone who is struggling with depression, anxiety, or feelings of worthlessness. Cannabidiol is a component of the plant *Cannabis sativa*, which probably now rings a bell for we are talking about the 'Marijuana plant.'

THC, or Δ^9-tetrahydrocannabinol, is the chemical in Marijuana that gets you high; there is no medical benefit to Marijuana or THC as a student.

Cannabidiol is a chemical constituent in Marijuana that is not psychoactive, yet in a scientific study released in 2016, we hear that

> CBD can be used for the "…treatment of motivational disorders such as drug addiction, anxiety, and depression…" (Zlebnik, Cheer)

There are a number of brands of CBD that are sold in smokeshops, though one that I would recommend is called "CBD Drip" which you can add to a 0mg nicotine liquid and then vape. If you are a smoker, you can add it to a 3mg or a 6mg nicotine liquid and vape it as usual.

Note: I am *not* talking about the type of CBD you must have a medical marijuana card to purchase, that type has THC in it. I am talking about the kind of CBD that *anyone* can purchase due to its 0mg THC content. This type of CBD is often extracted from industrial hemp, which is also used to make Hemp milk sold in grocery stores.

CORDYCEPS & REISHI

I discussed Cordyceps in detail in the first section of this book, but suffice it to say that if you take Cordyceps, they will help you feel better no matter what you currently feel like.

Reishi mushrooms are actually quite famous for their activation of certain parts of the immune system such that they are powerful against viruses. While they by no means can kill a virus themselves, they can provide valuable support to the immune system to help your body fight off viruses better.

It is this combination of both the energy-boosting effects of Cordyceps and the immune-boosting effects of Reishi mushrooms that makes this combination excellent against depression or feelings of despair.

I actually like a certain product by Host Defense called "CordyChi" which consists of equal parts of both Reishi mushroom and Cordyceps mushroom. I also am a big fan of NOW Foods Cordyceps and a good quality Reishi supplement. Many people have complained that NOW Foods is not well known for good quality products. I agree. However – somehow they did it right with their Cordyceps supplements, which never have failed me, even when other products have.

A final note on blending medicinal mushrooms: these things don't interact with many medications, so unless you are taking mammoth doses of medicinal mushrooms, these are generally some of the safest supplements you can take.

OVERCOME & PREVENT

ALCOHOL, DRUG-USE, AND CIGARETTES

I will explain some of the best ways to overcome hangovers and drug withdrawals, and I will explain methods you can use to help with your overall health.

TOBACCO

> ...the hazard to health arising from long-term vapour inhalation from the e-cigarettes available today is unlikely to exceed **5% of the harm from smoking tobacco**...
>
> April 2016 Statement by the Royal College of Physicians, U.K.

Smoking cigarettes is one of the worst things you can do for your health ever.

Keep in mind that nicotine is one of the world's deadliest poisons.

E-Cigarettes are the best way for you to switch from cigarettes to smoke-free nicotine.

An E-Cigarette has 3 parts: a battery (often called a mod), an atomizer (or cartomizer), and nicotine liquid.

> "Non-cancer risk analysis [for e-cigarettes] revealed 'No Significant Risk' [whereas cigarettes indicated] 'Significant Risk' ... Cancer risk analysis, no e-liquids exceeded the risk limits for either children or adults ... the tobacco smoke sample approached the risk limits for adult exposure" – 2012 Study

My recommendation is that you switch completely over to e-cigarettes, do not try to quit until you are ready, but eliminate tobacco completely.

My personal favorite e-cigarette company is found here, if you're new to e-cigarettes: http://www.smoktech.com/

ALCOHOL / HANGOVERS

My point in writing this book is to help people who are in college and attempting to do well in their studies. My point is *not* to be your parents or counselors. If you drink alcohol, either frequently or infrequently, that is your choice, I'm not going to go hardline and say quit drinking because that is quite frankly, your decision. Moreover, reversing alcohol-related brain damage is quite effective via the following supplementation routines.

If you drink frequently, or black out more than once a month: you should make it a priority to get to a campus alcohol and drug counselor. Each time you black out you kill over 100 million brain cells.

However, let's assume that you have no interest in a counselor, here is the best supplemental regimen for you to follow to make the best of this situation:
- → 1000mg Lion's Mane mushroom once per day
- → 500mg Milk Thistle once per day, in morning
- → 200mg Caffeine, twice daily
- → 400mg L-Theanine, twice daily (with caffeine)
- → 1 multivitamin per day
- → 3 Fish oil soft gels per day

If you drink alcohol frequently, but never black out: I would recommend:
- → 500mg Lion's Mane mushroom per day
- → 150mg Milk Thistle once per day, in morning
- → 1 multivitamin daily
- → 3 Fish oil soft gels per day

HEROIN, OPIATES, & HALLUCINOGENS (excluding Marijuana)

If you are addicted to these drugs, you need help. You need help right now.

Many people in your situation would benefit from one of two things: 1.) talking with the drug and alcohol counselor at your college and/or 2.) going to a local Narcotics Anonymous meeting. The folks in NA meetings are often half-way between life and death already and just need a support group to help them.

Heroin – For this one, you basically need professional help, and quickly. Your college health center/clinic, for example or even a local hospital.

Opiates/Painkillers – A legal substance known as Kratom is often sold in smokeshops and also online (but look for a high quality source). It is completely legal and while it is not an opioid, it activates the μ-opioid receptor agonist. It is very addictive, but if you are already addicted to something like painkillers, this is a better choice. You should absolutely seek help from a college health clinic if you are willing to, I urge you to do this.

Hallucinogens – The best advice I can give you, is stop while you are ahead. Continuing to use hallucinogens can lead to some incredible and amazing experiences. But it can also launch you into a lifetime of schizophrenia, terrible depression, or suicidal behavior, or even cause a reaction and kill you (since hallucinogens are illegal and thus manufactured in sub-par conditions). Also, get help from your college health clinic, they want to help.

SUICIDE ATTEMPT/THOUGHTS

The most important thing that you can do if you ever attempt to commit suicide or are thinking about it is to get help. But help can come in many forms, some supplemental, some external.

If you only wish to consider supplemental forms, L-Theanine is a good supplement for promoting relaxation and can calm you down so that you will think more straightforwardly.

St. John's Wort is a very powerful anti-depressant herb that will be invaluable to you as well. As suicide ends life, so therefore recommending something bad for your health is not an issue, smoking cigarettes or vaping is an excellent option as well, cigarettes being better, as it provides a powerful rush of energy and well-being feelings.

* * *

You also *need* some form of outside help as well. A significant other does not count, though you can consult with them. Ideally, you should speak with a doctor or psychologist, yet if you tell them of an active suicide plan, they *are required by law* to have you arrested by the police to keep you from harming yourself.

My recommendation for help is a religious authority figure. A priest, a pastor, a bishop – if you are not Christian, do not worry: an imam, a rabbi, a Buddhist leader etc., are all excellent choices as well. If you are an atheist, just pick one of the religious leaders above, approach them, and explain your situation to them. Because of their profession as a spiritual leader, they will help you.

RECREATIONAL MARIJUANA

> CBD …. [operates] at both CB_1 and CB_2 receptors …. Reducing the sudden withdrawal produced by abrupt cessation of cannabis use. (Copeland, Pokorski 2016)

Marijuana is addictive, and thus, you become dependent upon it and suffer withdrawals from it. **Taking a high quality CBD supplement (often vaporized through an e-cigarette, can reduce withdrawals from Marijuana smoking and make it easier to break this addiction.**

I know many people are convinced Marijuana is absolutely safe because their friends say so or because they want to believe that is true, so I selected three quotes from the Copeland/Pokorski article that provide a scientifically backed instead of emotionally backed information:

> …. 5% of the world's population who regularly use cannabis will develop a cannabis-use disorder, characterized by tolerance, craving, and a withdrawal syndrome. (Ramesh, Haney 2015)
>
> …. adolescent [read, those under 25 years of age] cannabis use can affect the prefrontal cortex and hippocampus, which are involved in attention, executive function, and memory, and may permanently impair adolescent neurocognitive functions. (Hooper, Woolley, De Bellis 2014)
>
> …. Cannabis use has frequently been linked to the development of mental illness, and while cross-sectional data frequently shows an association with anxiety and depression. (Grant 1995), (Chen, Wagner, Anthony 2002)

SUPPLEMENTS TO AVOID

In the following pages, I will detail the supplements I recommend you avoid.

OFF-LABEL MEDICAL MARIJUANA

> Heavy marijuana use is associated with residual neuropsychological effects even after a day of supervised abstinence from the drug. (Pope M.D., Yurgelun-Todd Ph.D.)

If you believe Marijuana use can help you focus, do well in your studies, relieve ADD/ADHD, or cure depression, you are very wrong.

According to NORML, the organization trying to get Marijuana legalized, the legitimate uses for Marijuana from a medical perspective are:

…. pain relief -- particularly of neuropathic pain (pain from nerve damage) -- nausea, spasticity, glaucoma, and movement disorders. Marijuana is also a powerful appetite stimulant, specifically for patients suffering from HIV, the AIDS wasting syndrome, or dementia. (norml.org Medical Marijuana)

Colorado recently made headlines due to a study that came out showing that hospitalizations due to the unsafe consumption of Marijuana (resulting in injury) had plummeted upon legalization recreationally, but that out-of-state residents hospitalizations had skyrocketed because they were not knowledgeable of how to indulge safely (Kim).

The bottom line is that you should not use Marijuana to help you with your studies, but if you have a doctor's orders to use it for a valid medical condition, do so, but do not think Marijuana use will help you study, its medical use is mostly limited to pain relief of various sorts.

L-DOPA / MUCUNA PRURIENS

Often recommended as a cure-all, L-Dopa (known as Velvet Bean, Mucuna Pruriens, and other names) is a dangerous supplement that works by boosting your dopamine levels. Dopamine is your pleasure hormone, but L-Dopa boosts it in an erratic fashion which can cause myriads of side-effects. For your health, never, ever, ever take L-Dopa. Doctors sometimes prescribe L-Dopa as a *last resort* in treatments for Parkinson's, but even then they are hesitant.

Do not take any supplement that contains L-Dopa, Mucuna Pruriens, or the Velvet Bean. It is a dangerous supplement.

Another problem with L-Dopa supplementation is that is quickly becomes steady in your body so you need to take more and more of it to get the same effect, and higher levels are increasingly dangerous to your health. Also, it is exceptionally addictive, probably due to its dopamine-affecting qualities, and if you are addicted to it, you will go through a literal hell before you stop going through withdrawals. Do not mess with this 'supplement,' it is crazy how prevalent it has become in various supplements.

MELATONIN

Melatonin is a supplement that is reaching a concerning new growth among college students due to the fact that it helps people who take way too much caffeine during the day quickly fall asleep at night.

Simply pop a melatonin capsule and off to sleep. Or so it seems. What happens, is melatonin is a supplement supplying your brain with a sleep hormone, but the problem is that your brain quickly becomes dependent on supplemental melatonin and thus without your nightly 'fix,' you are unable to fall asleep. If you miss too many nights of supplementation, you will start to suffer brain damage until your body adjusts to the lack of melatonin supplementation.

My suggestion is that you never use this supplement and that you instead take diphenhydramine (the generic for Benadryl) at 25mg – 75mg dose if you need help falling asleep instead of taking the so called 'all natural' melatonin supplement that will quickly make you addicted to it.

A very dangerous supplement to mess around with, I recommend staying well away from this.

SUPPLEMENTS TO FIGHT THE BIG 3: *THE COLD THE FLU THE STOMACH FLU*

Though often there is no 'cure' for these, and you just need to wait for them to naturally go away, there are supplements you can take that will speed up this process a LOT.

GARLIC

Garlic is your best natural form of medicine for *practically every* sickness or disease you can get, from the cold, flu, stomach flu, athletes foot, parasites from uncooked meat, inflamed wounds, to many other things..

> *Allicin, one of the active principles of freshly crust garlic .... [has] antibacterial activity .... Antifungal activity .... Antiparasitic activity .... Antiviral activity .... [the] antimicrobial effect of allicin is due to its chemical reaction with thiol groups of enzymes, e.g. alcohol dehydrogenase, ... Which can affect essential metabolism of cysteine proteinase activity ....* (Ankri, Mirelman 1999)

Thus, what the authors of this scientific paper are saying (which I will translate to a more normal sounding version of English) is that when you get a clove of garlic and crush it, you are releasing a powerful antiviral, antibiotic, antifungal, and antiparasitic chemical.

How to Use Garlic to Fight Colds/Flu?

Garlic supplements are not worth your money. You need to buy a bulb of garlic (the big round thing) and take two cloves from that bulb, peel them, and then crush them with a spoon. This is an essential step, for it releases this antimicrobial activity. Then, cover the crushed garlic with some honey, and swallow it, and drink some water too.

Your throat will feel an intense burning in it, but this is completely normal. If you are tempted to get garlic pills to avoid this feeling, remember: the pain is how you know it works, if you don't feel pain when you eat garlic, the garlic is dead and won't help you at all.

MILK THISTLE

Very importantly, you must make sure you use a supplement from a well-known company and make sure it is an extract and not just the plant itself. Milk thistle is a liver detox supplement with the main ingredient being Silybum marianum and with the sub-ingredients being Silymarin fractions isosilybinins A and B, silybinins A and B, silychristin and silydianin. That may sound like a mouthful, but it is very useful.

If you've ever heard of people who have eaten deadly poisonous mushrooms and been taken to the hospital and survived? Chances are, it's due to an intravenous injection of silibinins A and B from milk thistle. Have you ever met an alcoholic who tells you their liver is almost dead and that there is no hope since they cannot stop drinking? They are wrong: they can keep drinking and start supplementing with milk thistle (obviously, they will not live as long as if they quit drinking altogether but they will live a lot longer than with no milk thistle).

I recommend the Jarrow Formulas Milk Thistle 30:1 supplement, and take 3 pills each day, ideally every day. If you do this, you will notice some foul smells for the first week as your liver 'cleanses' itself. Milk Thistle activates your liver cells, and it one of the most useful immune system boosters known.

GREEN DRINK

A good quality green drink is one of your best supplements available to fight illnesses, for when you are sick, eating a huge plate of veggies is probably one of the last things on your mind.

There are a number of bad products on the market, so I'd recommend a green drink that has at least 500 reviews on amazon.com and has an average of 4.5 stars out of 5 or better. The Amazing Grass original superfood green drink is an excellent product, but there are many others, I mention this one because it is quite cheap and still effective.

The good thing about a green drink is that it gives you a portion of your recommended daily allowance of greens (which in all likelihood will be your only intake of greens). Green supplements are very useful when you are sick because they provide an alkalizing (or base) food into your diet and most of your other foods are more acidic (dairy products, meat products, grain products) so your body's natural balance of pH will be restored a little and will help you fight off sicknesses better.

COLLOIDAL SILVER

Colloidal silver is one of the few homeopathic medicines I will list in this book (probably the only one) since I believe that homeopathy is, to a large extent, a bogus form of medicine. However, colloidal silver is different. What makes colloidal silver so useful for is that it is a very small amount of silver which is toxic to humans in small amounts (but colloidal silver is extremely tiny amounts, not small amounts) but it is also lethal to germs and viruses (which are very small themselves).

I have seen a number of products that have 200-1000 PPM (parts per million) of colloidal silver. These are much less effective than products that have 10-30 PPM of silver in them. The reason is that you want a colloidal silver with the smallest particles of silver possible so that the silver can bind to germs and destroy them. I like Source Naturals colloidal silver, which can be found in many health food stores, and it is a well-known company, and well-respected.

Colloidal silver, due to its toxicity, should only be taken (generally a small portion mixed in a cup of water) throughout a sickness. When you swallow it, the silver binds to germs on the inside of your throat and kills them, thus weakening your cold or disease. It is a good secondary supplement to an excellent one like freshly crushed garlic.

SHIZANDRA

Shizandra is an herbal supplement you can buy that many people in the natural circles tend to promote for sexual energy and other properties. I personally believe that its most effective use is for fighting colds as it has a two-pronged approach to fighting colds: firstly, it reduces levels of stress in your body by making your brain get more activity and secondly it boosts your immune system which helps you fight the cold better.

Finding a quality Shizandra supplement is the main concern though, for there are many exceedingly cheap Shizandra supplements out there. If you are not interested in researching the different supplements available, I'd recommend the NOW Foods brand, which is a good overall brand of supplements, Dragon Herbs which is pricey but very high quality, or pretty much any Shizandra supplement that is sold in a good quality natural health store. Avoid supplements of any nature that are less than $5, for they are often heavily mixed with other 'safe' but unhelpful products like silica or gum.

Shizandra is a good secondary supplement, alongside a high quality antimicrobial agent like freshly crushed garlic.

PROBIOTICS

Probiotics are an essential daily supplement you should be taking because they help your gut health and also help your mental capacity because if your gut cannot digest food properly, your mind cannot get those nutrients either. But there are so many different probiotics to choose from, so how should you go about this process?

Probiotics are excellent for supplementation purposes, but I would recommend one with at least 5 Billion live probiotics in them because many are destroyed in your stomach acid so you need to take ones with a higher count of probiotics to be helpful.

Also, it is important to realize that probiotics are, essentially, 'healthy bacteria.' If you have recently taken antibiotics for an illness, guess what? Probiotics are bacteria, and the residual antibiotics in your system will kill the probiotics immediately, so if this is you, you'll want to take "Jarrow Formulas Sacharomyces Boulardii & MOS" which is designed specifically for people who have recently taken an antibiotic. Sacharomyces Boulardii is not a bacterial probiotic, instead it is a yeast (fungal) probiotic. Antibacterial medicine does nothing against funguses, and while funguses are generally thought of as a bad thing, this is a good one, in the same way that Cordyceps are a good fungus.

Why is a quality probiotic such a good thing? It gives your gut (which you put a lot of very nasty stuff into each day) a kind of daily 'first aid' so that your gut can help repair itself and keep you in optimal health.

EXAMPLE SUPPLEMENT 'STACKS'

I do encourage you to pick and choose from various herbs and supplements I discuss in this book, but if you would prefer me to recommend options for you, the following pages contain some example supplement stacks.

SUPPLEMENT 'STACK'

Now we have reached the end of our discussion of what herbs, activities, and supplements are important for college students who are seeking to maximize their potential, and now we have reached the time to discuss supplement stacks. A supplement stack is essentially a collection of supplements that work synergistically with each other to help you throughout your day.

An important element of a supplement stack is to make sure you have the main bases covered: energy, motivation, memory retention, and nutrition.

I highly encourage you to make up your own supplement stack based on your own personal needs, but the following example stacks will give you an opportunity to see what I suggest so that you can modify a supplement stack to meet your own needs.

Again, the important aspect of a supplement stack is to cover all bases: you cannot create a supplement stack that only helps your energy (such as a Caffeine and L-Theanine combination) because while you will be full of energy, you may be lacking in memory retention and what you read will simply not 'stick.' So it's important to thoroughly cover all bases when you are building your own supplement stack.

BARE MINIMUM STACK:

- 1 Multivitamin each day (look for a simple multivitamin with no added greens or other 'nutrients' just the basic vitamins and minerals.
- 2 quality fish oil soft gels each day.
- 1 Serving of a quality green food drink a day.

What makes this supplement stack useful?

It contains a multivitamin that gives you the essential nutrients and vitamins for your day. For example, iodine, which is important for your thyroid, is only obtainable from sources like kelp or iodized salt, but many lately have been going for regular salt and skipping the iodized version. A multivitamin will cover this deficiency and help you get your basic vitamins.

Fish oil is important for brain health, and two fish oil soft gels will help you boost your brain a little. They also are shown to provide a small boost for those fighting depression, which is yet another advantage of them, and if you don't have depression? Well, feeling a little better is never a bad thing, right?

And finally, a huge problem many college students face is poor nutrition, and a green food drink is vitally important as it is like your 'emergency rations' of greens, so that even if you go your entire day with burgers, pizza, and soda, you still get a little greens too.

HIGH QUALITY STACK #1:

- 1 Multivitamin daily
- 2 Fish Oils daily
- 1 Green Drink Each Morning/Night
- 2 NOW Foods Cordyceps Morning/Night
- 1 Host Defense Lion's Mane daily

What makes this supplement stack so useful?

It has your multivitamin, your fish oils, and your green drinks, which will build your health up mostly at a natural level. But it then also had Cordyceps which will give you a powerful boost in natural energy and motivation. Cordyceps are very famous throughout Traditional Chinese Medicine, and are one of the most famous of all adaptogenic herbs (or herbs that help your body on many different levels).

It also has a Lion's Mane mushroom supplement, which helps your brain in storing information. Many of the benefits of Lion's Mane do not show themselves within a month or two, so it is important to trust in the power of this supplement and keep taking it. Growing new brain cells is a lengthy process, but the benefits are excellent for college students.

HIGH QUALITY STACK #2:

- 1 Multivitamin daily
- 2 Fish Oils daily
- 1 Green Drink Each Morning/Night
- 1 Protein powder shake, with breakfast
- 1 Jarrow Formulas Milk Thistle before bed

What makes this supplement stack so useful?

I like to refer to this one as the 'detox from your day' supplement stack. College students who lead unhealthy lifestyles, be it cigarette smoking, alcohol consumption (of any amount – even a beer every couple of days), fast food, and similar, are in dire need of a detox and this supplement combo does just that: it gives your body the help It needs to detox: vitamins and fish oils, green drinks, protein powder for energy, and Milk Thistle for liver detox support.

Of course the individual ingredients in this stack can be heavily altered, and I encourage you to add or delete individual ingredients in this stack and make one of your own. This is the amazing thing about supplement stacks, you are always in control, and anything you take will essentially only help you since nearly every supplement only has good advantages.

HIGH QUALITY STACK #3:

- 1 Multivitamin daily
- 2 Fish Oils daily
- 1 Green Drink, with breakfast
- 6 NOW Foods Cordyceps, with breakfast
- >1000mg L-Theanine, with breakfast

What makes this supplement stack so useful?

This is a supplement stack that is essentially designed for college students who are tired frequently. It is not exactly for those who abuse their bodies through binge drinking but basically for those who are just tired. Schoolwork just is too much. Well, bad news schoolwork, with this supplement stack, a student can beat pretty much anything.

Cordyceps are a main component of this stack, and for good reason. Widely promoted for their mostly fictitious sexual boosting powers, these miracle supplements are one of the most elite of all adaptogenic supplements you can find: they promote energy, clear your mind and focus your mind, and stave off bad thoughts and depression. Mix this with L-Theanine and a few cups of coffee or tea and you get a mental powerhouse supplement with which you can conquer pretty much any obstacle. You may even consider adding 6 Cordyceps to your lunch meal as well, but I'd wait on that until you've used this stack for at least a month, Cordyceps are powerful energy boosters after all.

A WORD OF WARNING…
ON "DIETS FOR ENERGY"

I urge you to be very careful before you consider embarking on any special diet that is claimed to give you a huge boost in energy, for example:

- The Gluten Free Diet
- The Dairy Free Diet
- The Vegetarian/Vegan Diet
- The Paleo Diet
- And so on…

Often, these diets are very specific on what you are not allowed to eat and spent very little time explaining what you should eat to maintain peak health. For example, cutting grain out of your diet leaves you with a lot of protein and carbohydrates that you somehow need to start getting from another source. People come up with wild claims of all the health benefits from these diets, but unless you are willing to spend at least 2 hours each week researching herbal supplements and healthy recipes and nutrition, I urge you to eat the food your normally eat, whether it come from your dining commons or grocery store. Starting a new diet can have disastrous consequences for your health. The one exception to this is if your doctor or nutritionist recommends a diet, but even then ask specifically for things you should be eating to make up for nutrients you will no longer be getting from what you are not eating. Bottom line with diets: only start them if you *need* to instead of as an attempt to boost your energy.

IMPORTANT NOTE

Throughout this book, I am harshly critical of Marijuana use. The reason for this is that I believe in scientific data for the harms of Marijuana use relative to the cognitive and mental health aspects of the human mind. For a student, Marijuana smoking is akin to throwing your college tuition money in a fire and burning it to ashes.

There are specific medical situations for which I strongly support Medical Marijuana, but as you will notice, these are not cases that affect the vast majority of college students, so if you fall into one of the following categories, follow your doctor's orders.

Valid Reasons to Use Medical Marijuana:
> .... pain relief -- particularly of neuropathic pain (pain from nerve damage) -- nausea, spasticity, glaucoma, and movement disorders. Marijuana is also a powerful appetite stimulant, specifically for patients suffering from HIV, the AIDS wasting syndrome, or dementia. Emerging research suggests that marijuana's medicinal properties may protect the body against some types of malignant tumors and are neuroprotective. (norml.org)

To learn more about the medical applications for Marijuana, read the following link for more information on this: http://norml.org/marijuana/medical

WHAT ABOUT SUPPLEMENTS I DO NOT MENTION?

There are thousands upon thousands of supplements available for you to purchase. This book was written with the primary objective of helping students who are in college find a supplement regimen they can start following quickly and with minimal time to spend studying various herbs and supplements.

There are many worthwhile supplements you can be taking, for instance specialized vitamins from Methylfolate, to B-12 supplements to Vitamin D supplements, all three of which are very useful for brain health. There are myriads of others such as Coconut Oil, tea tree oil, and slippery elm bark extracts which each provide their own worthwhile uses. But I do not mention them. Why? If you were this interested in supplements, you would not be reading this book – you are reading this book because you want to know the most useful supplements and I'm giving you the most useful ones.

I encourage you to start reading about other supplements, but if you don't have the time, do not worry, the supplements I mention in this book are more than satisfactory – they are all excellent for the uses listed in this book, and with the energy they give you, you may indeed start learning more about supplements later on.

BAD & EXCELLENT BRANDS

Every supplement that is sold contains 100% pure ingredients, is absolutely beneficial for your health, and contains nutritious vitamins and minerals to support your mental integrity. Supplements are never mixed with fillers, contaminants such as heavy metals, and they never have ingredients other than those on the label.

We have all seen labels that say something along these lines, and I am here to explain to you how you can be sure that the supplement you are getting is high quality and will help you instead of not doing anything at all, or, worse, harming you. There are *many* more low quality supplements than there are good quality supplements, so it is very important to be able to distinguish the warning signs for low quality ones versus the good signs for the high quality ones.

Warning Signs for Low Quality Supplements:

- HIGH QUALITY (all capital letters)
- Less than 50 reviews on Amazon.com
- Poor English writing in many 5-star reviews
- Incorrect grammar in description of supplement
- Discontinued at a dollar store

Signs of a Good Quality Supplement:

- More than 50 reviews on Amazon.com
- Mixture of good *and* bad reviews on Amazon.com
- No outrageous claims (eg. cures fatigue!)
- Well-respected company (eg. NOW Foods)
- Sold at an *expensive* health food store

USEFUL LINKS

http://www.dragonherbs.com/
This is one of the websites I first read that made me very interested in supplements, especially in Traditional Chinese Medicine. It is filled with writings, history, facts, and recent discoveries. A very interesting website, but it's important to realize they are trying to sell their products, so watch out for 'advertorials' among the writings.

http://norml.org/
An interesting website that is pro-legalization of Marijuana. In this book, I recommend against recreational Marijuana use, but if you are interested in opposing viewpoints, this is an excellent resource.

http://www.maps.org/
A website for an organization studying the use of psychedelic drugs to treat PTSD and other serious medical conditions. Mostly an interesting site, but I caution against experimentation with these substances yourself, for outside of a clinically controlled area, they are highly dangerous.

http://peaknootropics.com/
This is the website I purchase nootropics from, it took me several weeks of sifting through sketchy looking websites to come across it, but it is a high quality resource for anything nootropic.

http://www.webmd.com/interaction-checker/default.htm
Useful resource to make sure your supplements do not interact in a harmful way with medicine.

BIBLIOGRAPHY

"Medical Use." NORML.org - Working to Reform Marijuana Laws. NORML.org, Web. 01 Aug. 2016. <http://norml.org/marijuana/medical>.

"Nicotine without Smoke: Tobacco Harm Reduction." *RCP London*. Royal College of Physicians, 27 Apr. 2016. Web. 15 July 2016. <https://www.rcplondon.ac.uk/projects/outputs/nicotine-without-smoke-tobacco-harm-reduction-0>.

Ankri, Serge, and David Mirelman. "Antimicrobial Properties of Allicin from Garlic." *Microbes and Infection*. Science Direct, Feb. 1999. Web. 31 July 2016.

Chen C-Y, Wagner FA, Anthony JC. Marijuana use and the risk of Major Depressive Episode. *Social psychiatry and psychiatric epidemiology*. 2002;37(5):199–206.

Copeland, Jan, and Izabella Pokorski. "Progress toward Pharmacotherapies for Cannabis-Use Disorder: An Evidence-Based Review." *Substance Abuse and Rehabilitation* 7 (2016): 41–53. PMC. Web. 2 Aug. 2016.

Grant BF. Comorbidity between DSM-IV drug use disorders and major depression: results of a national survey of adults. *Journal of Substance Abuse*. 1995;7(4):481–497.

Hooper SR, Woolley D, De Bellis MD. Intellectual, neurocognitive, and academic achievement in abstinent adolescents with cannabis use disorder. *Psychopharmacology*. 2014;231(8):1467–1477.

Huang, Tina L; Charyton, Christine. *Alternative Therapies in Health and Medicine* 14.5 (Sep/Oct 2008): 38-50.

Kim, Howard S. "Marijuana Tourism and Emergency Department Visits in Colorado — NEJM." *New England Journal of Medicine*. New England Journal of

Medicine, 25 Feb. 2016. Web. 19 July 2016. <http://www.nejm.org/doi/citedby/10.1056/NEJMc1515009#t=article#t=citedby>.

Lewis, Jason. http://www.youtube.com/playlist?list=PLveg0IEcZWN6mXfBEXLRyhbD9Y4Imvyu5

McAuley, TR, PK Hopke, J. Zhao, and S. Babaian. "Comparison of the Effects of E-cigarette Vapor and Cigarette Smoke on Indoor Air Quality." *National Center for Biotechnology Information*. U.S. National Library of Medicine, 24 Oct. 2012. Web. 18 July 2016. <http://www.ncbi.nlm.nih.gov/pubmed/23033998>.

Paterson, R. Russell M. "Cordyceps–A traditional Chinese medicine and another fungal therapeutic biofactory?." *Phytochemistry* 69.7 (2008): 1474. http://repositorium.sdum.uminho.pt/bitstream/1822/7896/1/Paterson_Cordyceps%255B1%255D.pdf

Pope HG, Jr, Yurgelun-Todd D. The Residual Cognitive Effects of Heavy Marijuana Use in College Students. *JAMA*. 1996;275(7):521-527. doi:10.1001/jama.1996.03530310027028.

Ramesh D, Haney M. Treatment of Cannabis Use Disorders. Textbook of Addiction Treatment: International Perspectives. 2015:367–380.<http://www.sciencedirect.com/science/article/pii/S1286457999800033>.

Unnatural Vegan. "Why I'm a Pro-GMO Vegan (and 9 Gmo Myths Dispelled)." YouTube. YouTube, 11 Feb. 2015. Web. 15 July 2016. <https://www.youtube.com/watch?v=aA4I-WRu_s0>.

Winnicka, K; Tomasiak, M; Bielawska, A (2005). "Piracetam--an old drug with novel properties?".

Acta poloniae pharmaceutica 62 (5): 405–9. PMID 16459490.

Zlebnik, Natalie E., and Joseph F. Cheer. "Beyond the CB1 Receptor: Is Cannabidiol the Answer for Disorders of Motivation?" *Annu. Rev. Neurosci. Annual Review of Neuroscience* 39.1 (2015): Reviews in Advance. Reviews in Advance, 12 Feb. 2016. Web. 19 July 2016.
<http://www.cheerlab.org/pdf/zlebnik.pdf>.

ABOUT THE AUTHOR

For several years, I have been interested in natural health, supplements, and herbal medicine, especially Traditional Chinese Medicine and Nootropics. I currently live in Davis, California and am a graduate from the University of California, Davis, with a major in English and emphases in both Literature, Criticism, and Theory as well as Creative Writing. I enjoy reading about Traditional Chinese Medicine, current news, reading new books, and exercising in my spare time.

Philosophy of this Book:
I also hold the firm belief that Western Medicine is a *good* thing and thus if you want to read a book that trash-talks prescription medicines, this is not the book for you. I believe in a comprehensive form of supplementation: valuable things that you can take to improve your health in addition to regular visits to a doctor, a good health program including exercise, hygiene, and diet, and a good group of friends. Supplementation is just what it is named for: something that supplements something else.

www.ingramcontent.com/pod-product-compliance
Lightning Source LLC
Chambersburg PA
CBHW070403190526
45169CB00003B/1091